UNDERSTANDING
VITAMIN D
AND BENEFITS

A Guide To Science, Sources, Depth Exploration And Its Key Points For Optimal Health

DR. LACEY MICHELLE

Disclaimer:

The information provided in this book is for general informational purposes only and is not intended as medical advice.

Readers are encouraged to consult with a qualified healthcare professional for any health concerns or questions.

The author of this book is not affiliated with any individual, website, organization, or products mentioned within.

This book does not endorse or promote any specific brands, services, or external entities. Any references made are purely for illustrative purposes and should not be construed as endorsements.

Readers are responsible for their own decisions and should conduct their own research before making any health-related choices.

Any liability resulting from the use of this information, whether direct or indirect, is disclaimed by the author and publisher.

Contents

CHAPTER ONE

The Basics of Vitamin D

Vitamin D is a fat-soluble vitamin that plays a crucial role in various physiological processes within the human body.

It is essential for the maintenance of strong bones and teeth, as it helps the body absorb calcium and phosphorus from the food we consume.

Vitamin D also contributes to the immune system's functioning, muscle function, and overall cell growth and development. This multifaceted vitamin is unique because our bodies can synthesize it when exposed to sunlight, making it distinct from most other vitamins that primarily come from dietary sources.

Vitamin D is not a single compound but rather a group of fat-soluble secosteroids, with two primary forms that are most important for human health: vitamin D2 (ergocalciferol) and vitamin D3 (cholecalciferol).

Vitamin D2 is mainly found in plant-based sources and supplements, while vitamin D3 is synthesized by the skin upon exposure to sunlight and is also present in animal-derived sources like fish, eggs, and dairy products.

Both forms can be converted in the body to the biologically active form, calcitriol, which regulates calcium and phosphorus absorption in the intestines.

Types Of Vitamin D

As mentioned, there are two primary types of vitamin D: D2 and D3. Vitamin D2 is primarily obtained from plant-based sources, such as fortified foods and some mushrooms. However, it is generally less effective at raising blood levels of the active form of vitamin D compared to vitamin D3.

 Vitamin D3 is synthesized in the skin when exposed to ultraviolet B (UVB) sunlight and is also found in animal-derived sources, making it a more potent and effective source of vitamin D for the human body.

Additionally, there are several synthetic forms of vitamin D used in supplements and fortified foods, but their efficacy may vary.

Sources Of Vitamin D

Vitamin D can be obtained through various dietary sources and sun exposure. Dietary sources include fatty fish like salmon, mackerel, and tuna, egg yolks, fortified dairy products, and some fortified plant-based foods like cereals and plant-based milk alternatives. However, it can be challenging to get enough vitamin D from diet alone, and for this reason, sunlight plays a significant role in maintaining optimal vitamin D levels. When our skin is exposed to UVB radiation from the sun, it synthesizes vitamin D3, making sunlight a primary natural source of this essential vitamin.

The Role Of Sunlight In Vitamin D Production

Sunlight, specifically ultraviolet B (UVB) rays, is a critical factor in the synthesis of vitamin D within the human body.

When UVB rays interact with the cholesterol present in our skin, it triggers a chemical reaction that results in the formation of cholecalciferol, the precursor of active vitamin D.

The efficiency of this process depends on various factors, including geographical location, time of day, season, skin pigmentation, and the use of sunscreen. While sunlight exposure is essential for vitamin D synthesis, it's important to strike a balance to prevent overexposure and skin damage.

Recommended Dietary Allowances (Rdas) And Adequate Intake

The recommended daily intake of vitamin D varies based on factors such as age, sex, and life stage.

The Recommended Dietary Allowances (RDAs) and Adequate Intake (AI) values provide guidelines for the optimal daily vitamin D intake to maintain health.

For infants, children, and adults, the RDAs are typically expressed in International Units

(IUs), which measure the biological activity of the vitamin.

These recommendations take into account the vitamin D obtained from both dietary sources and sunlight exposure. Adequate intake levels are established when there is insufficient scientific evidence to establish an RDA.

vitamin D is a vital nutrient for human health, primarily known for its role in calcium and phosphorus metabolism, bone health, and immune system support.

It exists in multiple forms, with vitamin D2 and D3 being the most significant for human well-being. While dietary sources are essential for meeting vitamin D requirements, sunlight is a natural and crucial factor in its synthesis.

Understanding the various types of vitamin D and the role of sunlight in its production, along with following recommended intake guidelines, is vital for maintaining overall health and preventing deficiency-related issues.

CHAPTER TWO

Health Benefits Of Vitamin D

Vitamin D is a crucial fat-soluble vitamin that plays a pivotal role in various physiological processes within the human body. It is primarily obtained through exposure to sunlight and dietary sources.

This vitamin has a significant impact on a range of health aspects, including bone health, immune system support, cardiovascular health, mental health, cancer prevention, autoimmune disorders, and skin health. Each of these facets is influenced by the intricate mechanisms through which vitamin D operates.

Vitamin D And Bone Health

One of the most well-known and established functions of vitamin D is its essential role in maintaining optimal bone health.

It facilitates the absorption of calcium and phosphorus in the intestine, ensuring that these minerals are available for bone mineralization.

Vitamin D deficiency can lead to weakened bones and conditions like rickets in children and osteoporosis in adults.

Adequate vitamin D levels are crucial for bone density and the prevention of fractures.

Vitamin D And Immune System Support

Vitamin D plays a critical role in supporting the immune system.

It helps regulate both the innate and adaptive immune responses, aiding the body in defending against pathogens. Adequate vitamin D levels can enhance the body's ability to fight infections and reduce the risk of autoimmune diseases. There is ongoing research into the potential role of vitamin D in preventing and managing conditions like influenza and autoimmune disorders.

Vitamin D and Cardiovascular Health

Emerging evidence suggests that vitamin D may contribute to cardiovascular health. It is believed to influence blood pressure regulation and the health of the endothelium, the inner lining of blood vessels. Maintaining optimal levels of vitamin D may reduce the risk of heart disease and improve overall cardiovascular well-being. However, more research is needed to establish the exact mechanisms and benefits.

Vitamin D And Mental Health

Vitamin D is associated with mental health, as receptors for this vitamin are found in various regions of the brain. Research has indicated that low vitamin D levels may be linked to an increased risk of mood disorders such as depression and seasonal affective disorder. The mechanisms behind this relationship are still being explored, but vitamin D supplementation is considered a potential component of mental health support.

Vitamin D And Cancer Prevention

There is a growing body of research exploring the link between vitamin D and cancer prevention. Some studies have suggested that adequate vitamin D levels may reduce the risk of certain types of cancer, including breast, colon, and prostate cancer.

The exact mechanisms by which vitamin D impacts cancer prevention are multifaceted and continue to be the subject of active investigation.

Vitamin D And Autoimmune Disorders

Autoimmune disorders occur when the immune system mistakenly targets the body's tissues. Vitamin D has immunomodulatory properties that can help regulate immune responses.

Research has shown that maintaining sufficient levels of vitamin D may be associated with a reduced risk of autoimmune diseases like multiple sclerosis, rheumatoid arthritis, and type diabetes. However, the role of vitamin D in autoimmune disorders is complex, and further studies are needed to fully understand its implications.

CHAPTER THREE

Vitamin D And Skin Health

Skin is the body's primary source of vitamin D, as it synthesizes the vitamin when exposed to sunlight.

However, excessive sun exposure without protection can lead to skin damage and an increased risk of skin cancer.

Maintaining a balance between sun exposure and skin protection is essential for both vitamin D production and skin health. Additionally, vitamin D may play a role in skin conditions such as psoriasis.

vitamin D is a versatile and crucial vitamin that exerts a wide range of health benefits. It plays a fundamental role in bone health, immune system support, cardiovascular well-being, mental health, cancer prevention, autoimmune disorders, and even skin health. While vitamin D can be obtained through sunlight and diet, supplementation is often necessary to maintain optimal levels, especially in regions with limited sunlight or for individuals with specific health conditions. Ongoing research continues to shed light on the many ways vitamin D contributes to our overall health and well-being.

Vitamin D Deficiency

Vitamin D is an essential fat-soluble vitamin that plays a crucial role in various physiological processes in the human body. Its primary function is to regulate calcium and phosphorus absorption in the intestines, ensuring the maintenance of healthy bones and teeth. A deficiency in vitamin D can lead to a wide range of health problems, making it important to understand the causes, symptoms, and risk factors associated with this condition.

Causes of Vitamin D Deficiency

Several factors can contribute to a deficiency in vitamin D. One of the primary reasons is inadequate sun exposure. Vitamin D is often referred to as the "sunshine vitamin" because our skin produces it when exposed to sunlight.

Therefore, people who live in regions with limited sunlight or those who spend most of their time indoors are at a higher risk of deficiency. Additionally, the use of sunscreen, which blocks the UVB rays necessary for vitamin D synthesis, can also hinder its production.

Dietary factors can also lead to vitamin D deficiency. Some individuals may not consume enough foods rich in vitamin D, such as fatty fish (e.g., salmon, mackerel), fortified dairy products, and egg yolks. Vegan or vegetarian diets that lack animal-based products may also result in lower vitamin D intake.

Furthermore, certain medical conditions, like celiac disease, Crohn's disease, or kidney problems, can interfere with the body's ability to absorb or metabolize vitamin D.

Common Symptoms Of Vitamin D Deficiency

Recognizing the symptoms of vitamin D deficiency is essential for timely diagnosis and intervention. Some common symptoms include:

Bone Pain: Vitamin D deficiency can lead to bone and muscle pain, as it affects calcium absorption, which is essential for bone health.

Muscle Weakness: Weakness in the muscles can occur due to insufficient vitamin D, making everyday activities more challenging.

Fatigue: People with vitamin D deficiency often experience unexplained fatigue and a general sense of tiredness.

Mood Changes: There is evidence to suggest a link between low vitamin D levels and mood disorders, such as depression and seasonal affective disorder (SAD).

Impaired Wound Healing: Vitamin D plays a role in the body's immune response and wound healing, so deficiencies can slow down the healing process.

Hair Loss: In some cases, hair loss or excessive hair shedding can be associated with a lack of vitamin D.

Frequent Illness: A weakened immune system due to vitamin D deficiency may result in a higher susceptibility to infections.

Groups At Risk For Vitamin D Deficiency
Certain population groups are more susceptible to vitamin D deficiency. These include:

Elderly Individuals: Aging skin produces less vitamin D, and older people often have limited sun exposure, which can put them at higher risk.

People with Darker Skin: Melanin, the pigment responsible for skin color, reduces the body's ability to produce vitamin D from sunlight. As a result, individuals with darker skin may need more sun exposure to maintain adequate levels.

Infants and Young Children: Babies who are exclusively breastfed and not receiving vitamin D supplementation are at risk, as breast milk alone may not provide enough vitamin D.

Individuals with Limited Sun Exposure: Those who live in regions with long winters, work indoors, or cover most of their skin for cultural or religious reasons are at risk of deficiency.

Obese Individuals: Excess body fat can sequester vitamin D, making it less available for the body to use.

Diagnosing Vitamin D Deficiency

Diagnosing vitamin D deficiency typically involves a blood test to measure the levels of

25-hydroxyvitamin D in the bloodstream. The normal range for vitamin D levels can vary, but typically, a level below 20 nanograms per milliliter (ng/mL) is considered deficient. Levels between 20-30 ng/mL may be classified as insufficient, while optimal levels are generally considered to be above 30 ng/mL.

vitamin D deficiency is a common health concern with various causes, symptoms, and risk factors.

Recognizing the signs and addressing the deficiency through increased sun exposure, dietary changes, and supplements when necessary can help maintain overall health and prevent the associated health issues.

CHAPTER FOUR

Using Vitamin D Supplements:

Vitamin D is an essential nutrient that plays a crucial role in maintaining overall health. While the primary source of vitamin D is sunlight exposure, many individuals may require vitamin D supplements to meet their daily needs. This is particularly important for those who have limited sun exposure, live in regions with minimal sunlight, or have specific health conditions that hinder their ability to produce or absorb vitamin D efficiently. In this context, understanding how to use vitamin D supplements effectively is essential for ensuring optimal health and well-being.

Types Of Vitamin D Supplements:

There are two primary forms of vitamin D supplements available in the market: vitamin

D2 (ergocalciferol) and vitamin D3 (cholecalciferol). Vitamin D3 is the most bioactive form and is typically recommended over vitamin D2, as it raises blood levels of vitamin D more effectively. It is synthesized from cholesterol and is the form that our skin produces when exposed to UVB sunlight. Vitamin D3 supplements are often derived from animal sources like lanolin or fish oil, making them the preferred choice for many. On the other hand, vitamin D2 is derived from plant sources and may not be as potent in raising vitamin D levels in the body.

Choosing The Right Vitamin D Supplement:

When selecting a vitamin D supplement, it's important to consider factors such as the form of vitamin D, the source of the supplement, and additional ingredients. As previously mentioned, vitamin D3 is generally the preferred choice for supplementation. Additionally, the source of the supplement may matter to individuals following specific dietary restrictions (e.g., vegans may prefer plant-based vitamin D2 supplements).

Check the label for additional ingredients and fillers, as some supplements may contain unnecessary additives that you may want to avoid. Always opt for reputable brands and look for supplements with third-party testing to ensure quality and purity.

Dosage And Safety Guidelines:

The appropriate dosage of vitamin D supplements can vary widely depending on individual factors such as age, sex, weight, and existing health conditions. It is advisable to consult with a healthcare professional to determine the correct dosage for your specific needs. In general, the Recommended Dietary Allowance (RDA) for vitamin D varies by age and life stage, but it typically ranges from 400 to 800 international units (IU) per day.

However, individuals with deficiency or certain health issues may require higher doses, which should be carefully monitored by a healthcare provider.

It's important to note that excessive vitamin D intake can lead to toxicity, resulting in symptoms like nausea, vomiting, and hypercalcemia.

Thus, it is crucial to follow dosage recommendations and undergo periodic blood tests to monitor your vitamin D levels while taking supplements.

Interactions And Side Effects:

Vitamin D supplements can interact with other medications and nutrients. For example, certain medications like corticosteroids, weight loss drugs, and anticonvulsants can interfere with vitamin D metabolism. In addition, excessive calcium intake alongside vitamin D supplementation can lead to kidney stones. Therefore, if you are taking other medications or have specific medical conditions, it's essential to consult with a healthcare professional to ensure there are no adverse interactions.

Common side effects of vitamin D supplementation are typically mild and include gastrointestinal discomfort, constipation, and dry mouth. These side effects can often be mitigated by taking the supplement with food or adjusting the timing of intake.

Monitoring Your Vitamin D Levels: Regular monitoring of your vitamin D levels is crucial to ensure that you are taking the correct dosage and avoiding both deficiency and toxicity.

A simple blood test can measure your serum 25-hydroxyvitamin D levels, which reflect your overall vitamin D status. Your healthcare provider can interpret the results and adjust your supplement dosage accordingly.

It's particularly important for individuals who have medical conditions affecting vitamin D absorption or metabolism, such as celiac disease, Crohn's disease, or kidney disorders.

vitamin D supplements can be a valuable tool in maintaining optimal health, especially for those with limited sun exposure or specific health conditions.

Choosing the right type of supplement, following appropriate dosage guidelines, considering potential interactions and side effects, and regularly monitoring your vitamin D levels are all essential aspects of using vitamin D supplements effectively to support your overall well-being. Always consult with a healthcare professional for personalized guidance on vitamin D supplementation.

CHAPTER FIVE

Vitamin D And Special Populations

Vitamin D, often referred to as the "sunshine vitamin," is a crucial nutrient that plays a significant role in various physiological functions within the human body.

While it can be synthesized in the skin upon exposure to sunlight, dietary supplementation becomes necessary for specific population groups, including infants and children, pregnant and breastfeeding women, the elderly, and athletes or active individuals, to meet their unique nutritional requirements.

In this discussion, we'll delve into the role of vitamin D within each of these special populations.

Vitamin D is particularly essential for infants and children as it is vital for the development of strong bones and overall growth.

A deficiency in vitamin D during childhood can lead to rickets, a condition characterized by weakened and deformed bones. Infants who are exclusively breastfed may be at a higher risk of vitamin D deficiency since human milk contains relatively low levels of this vitamin.

To address this, pediatricians often recommend vitamin D supplementation for infants, typically starting shortly after birth.

Supplementation guidelines can vary by region and specific pediatric recommendations, but generally, a daily vitamin D supplement is provided to infants in their first year of life. This supplementation helps ensure that they receive the necessary vitamin D for proper bone mineralization and overall health.

Additionally, vitamin D supports the immune system and may have a role in reducing the risk of certain chronic diseases, which is of concern in today's society with the increasing prevalence of childhood obesity.

Vitamin D For Pregnant And Breastfeeding Women

Pregnant and breastfeeding women have unique vitamin D requirements as they must support both their health and the development of the fetus or infant. Vitamin D plays a crucial role in calcium absorption, which is vital for maintaining healthy bones in both the mother and the developing baby. A deficiency in this vitamin during pregnancy can lead to complications such as gestational diabetes and preeclampsia, as well as adverse outcomes for the baby.

While it is possible to meet some of the vitamin D needs through sun exposure, the use of sunscreen and limited outdoor activities can hinder this natural process. Therefore, pregnant and breastfeeding women are often advised to take vitamin D supplements to ensure they meet their recommended intake levels. The specific dosage should be determined in consultation with a healthcare provider, as individual needs can vary.

Vitamin D For The Elderly

The elderly population is particularly susceptible to vitamin D deficiency due to various factors, including decreased skin synthesis of vitamin D, reduced dietary intake, and limited sun exposure. This deficiency can have serious health consequences, including increased risk of osteoporosis, fractures, and muscle weakness. Ensuring adequate vitamin D levels in the elderly is critical for maintaining bone health and overall well-being.

Supplementation is often recommended for older individuals, especially those living in nursing homes or who have limited mobility. Adequate vitamin D intake can help reduce the risk of falls and fractures, which are significant concerns for the elderly population. Furthermore, vitamin D has been linked to cognitive health and immune function in older adults, making it even more crucial for this demographic.

Vitamin D For Athletes And Active Individuals

Active individuals and athletes also require optimal vitamin D levels to support their physical performance and overall health. Vitamin D is known to play a role in muscle function, which is of particular importance for athletes. Insufficient vitamin D levels can lead to muscle weakness, reduced endurance, and an increased risk of injuries.

While athletes often spend a considerable amount of time outdoors, factors like geographical location, weather, and the use of sunscreen can still impede the body's ability to synthesize sufficient vitamin D from sunlight.

As a result, many athletes, especially those training indoors or in less sunny climates, may benefit from vitamin D supplementation.

Proper vitamin D levels can aid in muscle recovery, enhance athletic performance, and reduce the risk of stress fractures and other musculoskeletal issues.

Vitamin D is a critical nutrient for individuals across various life stages and lifestyles. Supplementation is often necessary to meet the unique requirements of special populations such as infants and children, pregnant and breastfeeding women, the elderly, and athletes or active individuals. It is imperative for healthcare providers and individuals to be aware of these specific needs and to tailor vitamin D supplementation accordingly to promote optimal health and well-being.

CHAPTER SIX

The Future Of Vitamin D Research

Vitamin D, a fat-soluble vitamin, has long been recognized for its essential role in maintaining bone health, but recent research has expanded our understanding of its multifaceted functions within the body.

As we delve into the future of Vitamin D research, it becomes clear that this vital nutrient is far more than just a bone-supporting agent. Ongoing studies and emerging research trends promise to unlock its full potential in promoting overall health and well-being.

Ongoing Studies And Research Trends

In recent years, there has been a surge in Vitamin D research, leading to new insights and applications. One of the most notable trends in this area is the exploration of the relationship between Vitamin D and various chronic diseases. Epidemiological studies have linked Vitamin D deficiency to a higher risk of conditions such as cardiovascular disease, autoimmune disorders, diabetes, and even some types of cancer. These findings have sparked ongoing investigations into the potential preventive and therapeutic roles of Vitamin D in these diseases.

Moreover, research is increasingly focusing on the interaction between Vitamin D and the immune system. Studies have shown that Vitamin D plays a crucial role in modulating the immune response, which has significant implications for conditions related to immune dysfunction, such as allergies and autoimmune diseases. The ability of Vitamin D to enhance the body's defense mechanisms against infections is a particularly intriguing avenue of exploration in the context of the ongoing global health challenges, including the COVID-19 pandemic.

Beyond health, research is expanding into the effects of Vitamin D on various physiological processes. Recent studies have suggested a potential link between Vitamin D and mood disorders, particularly depression. Although the exact mechanisms are not fully understood, there is growing interest in exploring how Vitamin D supplementation may help improve mental well-being, opening up new avenues for research in the field of psychology and psychiatry.

Additionally, research on Vitamin D metabolism and its genetic variations is another promising area of study. Understanding the genetic factors that influence how individuals metabolize and respond to Vitamin D could lead to personalized recommendations for supplementation, optimizing health outcomes based on an individual's genetic makeup.

Potential New Applications Of Vitamin D
The expanding body of research on Vitamin D is also leading to the identification of potential new applications for this versatile nutrient. One of the most exciting areas is the potential for Vitamin D in preventing and managing autoimmune diseases. Multiple sclerosis, rheumatoid arthritis, and type 1 diabetes are examples of conditions where Vitamin D's immunomodulatory properties could be harnessed to improve patient outcomes.

Vitamin D's role in maintaining musculoskeletal health is well-established, but it's now being explored for its impact on athletic performance and muscle function. Athletes and fitness enthusiasts are increasingly turning to Vitamin D supplementation to potentially enhance their physical performance and recovery.

Skin conditions such as psoriasis and atopic dermatitis may also benefit from Vitamin D interventions. Topical Vitamin D analogs have shown promise in managing these conditions, with ongoing research aiming to refine treatment protocols and explore their long-term effects.

Conclusion

In the realm of cancer research, the potential for Vitamin D as a complementary therapy in cancer prevention and treatment is generating considerable interest. Although more research is needed to fully establish its efficacy, early findings indicate that Vitamin

D may have a role to play in inhibiting tumor growth and enhancing the outcomes of cancer therapies.

the future of Vitamin D research is poised for continued growth and discovery.

Ongoing studies are uncovering its roles in various physiological processes and diseases while emerging research trends are expanding our understanding of this essential nutrient. With the potential new applications of Vitamin D in disease prevention, mental health, genetics, and beyond, Vitamin D is likely to continue playing a pivotal role in the quest for improved health and well-being in the years to come.

www.ingramcontent.com/pod-product-compliance
Lightning Source LLC
Chambersburg PA
CBHW060815260726

48660CB00002B/958